STOP MISSI

DON'T LOOK BACK IN REGRET

You Only Live Once
Make The Most of It

Kent Reynolds

Table of Contents

Chapter 1: There's No Time for Regrets 6

Chapter 2: How To Not Live Your Life In Regret 9

Chapter 3: 10 Habits That Will Make Your Life Better...........................16

Chapter 4: *How To Have Proper Time Management* 20

Chapter 5: 7 Ways To Stop Overthinking And Relieve Stress 23

Chapter 6: Discovering Your Strengths and Weaknesses 27

Chapter 7: How Much Is Your Time Really Worth? 30

Chapter 8: The Keys To Happiness 32

Chapter 9: 5 Ways To Deal with Personal Feelings of Inferiority 34

Chapter 10: Happy People Stay Present 37

Chapter 11: *Productivity Mistake: Being in Motion Vs. Taking Action*...........39

Chapter 12: Happy People Don't Sweat the Small Stuff. 42

Chapter 13: *Motivation With Good Feelings*.......................................45

Chapter 14: *7 Ways To Attract Happiness* 48

Chapter 15: Trust The Process 52

Chapter 16: Stop Being a Slave To Old Beliefs.....................................54

Chapter 17: Deal With Your Fears Now 57

Chapter 18: Bounce Back From Failure..61

Chapter 19: How To Stop Procrastinating..64

Chapter 20: *Stop Wasting Time on the Details and Commit to the Fundamentals* 68

Chapter 21: 16 Steps To Stop Feeling Like Shit 71

Chapter 22: 10 Habits of Amancio Ortega Gaona 75

Chapter 23: *Treat Failure Like A Scientist*...79

Chapter 24: *Make Your Life Better By Saying 'Thank You'*.................82

Chapter 25: 10 Habits Of Happy People...85

Chapter 26: Happy People are Okay with Not Being Okay................... 89
Chapter 27: 6 Ways To Attract Anything You Want In Life 91
Chapter 28: Saying Yes To Things 95
Chapter 29: How To Stop Being A Narcissist 100
Chapter 30: 10 Habits of Mukesh Ambani 103
Chapter 31: When It Is Time To Let Go and Move On (Career) 107
Chapter 32: How To Improve Your Communication Skills 110
Chapter 33: 9 Signs You're Feeling Insecure About a Relationship ... 113
Chapter 34: 6 Ways To Master Your Emotions 118

Chapter 1:
There's No Time for Regrets

Regret. Guilt. Shame.

These are three of the darkest emotions any human will ever experience. We all feel these things at different points in our lives, especially after making a "bad" decision. There are certain situations some of us would rewind (or delete) if we could. The reality is, however, there is an infinite number of reasons we should never regret any of the decisions we make in our lives.

Here are 7 of them:

1. Every decision allows you to take credit for creating your own life.

Decisions are not always the result of thoughtful contemplation. Some of them are made on impulse alone. Regardless of the decision, when you made it, it was something you wanted, or you would not have done it (unless someone was pointing a gun at your head).

Be willing to own the decisions you make. Be accountable for them. Take responsibility and accept them.

2. By making any decision involving your heart, you have the chance to create more love in the world by spreading yours.

Your love is a gift.

Once you decide to love, do it without reservation. By fully giving of yourself, you expand your ability to express and receive love. You have added to the goodness of our universe by revealing your heart to it.

3. By experiencing the disappointment that might come with a decision's outcome, you can propel yourself to a new level of emotional evolution.

You aren't doing yourself any favors when you try to save yourself from disappointment. Disappointment provides you with an opportunity to redefine your experiences in life. By refining your reframing skills, you increase your resilience.

4. "Bad" decisions are your opportunity to master the art of self-forgiveness.

When you make a "bad" decision, *you* are the person who is usually the hardest on yourself. Before you can accept the consequences of your decision and move on, you must forgive yourself. You won't always make perfect choices in your life. Acknowledge the beauty in your human imperfection, then move forward and on.

5. Because of the occasional misstep, you enable yourself to live a Technicolor life.

Anger. Joy. Sadness.

These emotions add pigment to your life. Without these things, you would feel soulless. Your life would be black and white.

Make your decisions with gusto. Breathe with fire. You are here to live in color.

6. Your ability to make a decision is an opportunity to exercise the freedom that is your birthright.

How would you feel if you had no say in those decisions concerning your life? Would you feel powerless? Restricted? Suffocated?

Now, focus on what it feels like to make the decisions you want to make. What do you feel? Freedom? Liberty? Independence?

What feelings do you *want* to feel Freedom. Liberty. Independence. As luck would have it, the freedom you want is yours. Be thankful for it in every decision you make, "good" or "bad."

7. When you decide to result in ugly aftermath, you refine what you *do* want in your life.

It's often impossible to know what you want until you experience what you don't want. With every decision, you will experience consequences. Use those outcomes as a jumping-off point to something different (and better) in your future.

Chapter 2:
How To Not Live Your Life In Regret

Today we're going to talk about a simple yet profound topic that I hope will awaken something in you today if you have been sleeping on the wheel of your life. I hope that with this video, I can help you to stop wasting precious time and to keep doing the things that you've always said you wanted to do right now this day. Not tomorrow, but today.

Before we go any further, I want you to write down the things you wish to accomplish before you die. It can be as small as saying I love you to your mom and dad, to something bigger like quitting your job to find something you are passionate about, to leisurely things such as travelling to XXX countries by whatever age. To things such as picking up an instrument that you've always wanted to learn but told yourself you just didn't have the time or that you wont be able to do it, or other things such as making new friends, starting a family, or literally anything under the sun.

I want you to write these things down no matter how big or small, and make them a bucket list of sorts. Many people think that a bucket list is always a leisure thing, but many a times, our bucket list could be more significant in that it is something that we don't just want to do, but need to do.

We may not fill every single thing on that bucket list, but if we can even do half of them, we can say that at least we have tried and we don't regret a single thing. The fact that we attempted is sometimes good enough, it is definitely better than not even trying and living with the guilt of "what if".

Now that we have got this list down. I'm going to jump right into the one thing that will help us put all of this into perspective. And help us truly see what matters at the top of our list. And I think you will be surprised that it may not have anything to do with travel and leisure, but it is the personal goals that we have been putting off.

Are you ready for it?

I want you to close your eyes right now. Find a quiet space where no one will disturb you for the next 5-10mins. I want you to pause this video if you need to at any one point. And I want you to visualise yourself at your deathbed, at the end of your life, whether you see yourself being 80, 90, 100, or even 60 or 70, if you feel that maybe u dont see yourself living a long life. Whatever it may be, I want you to picture yourself in your last moments.

Now I want you to ask yourself, what do you regret not having done in your 20s, 30s, and 40s. What is that one thing that you just couldn't live with yourself having not done, and what that greatest regret may be. Was it not committing your life to helping others, was it not pursuing your passion? Was it not being a good father, mother, child, friend, lover?

What is it? Who do you see around you? Are there any friends that are there to see you off? Are there any family members, cousins, loved ones there? Or have you not been a good person that none of them are there to see you? Are you lonely or surrounded my love? Are you happy that you've kept your word and done the things you said you would? Or do you regret not trying?

Do you feel like your heart is full because you have conquered every experience that life has to offer? Or do you regret not spending enough time outside seeing the world for what it truly is? Do you regret not moving to a country that you said you would one day, and just lived to see people live their best lives vicariously through Instagram and Facebook and YouTube? I want you to be as honest as you can with yourself about your current actions and project them forward into the future. Are they going to bring about the kind of peace that you would feel at the end of your life knowing you've done everything you possibly can and without regret?

Take some time to think about the things I said and see if you can paint a vivid picture of what they is like. Did you commit to eating healthily that you can see yourself living to a ripe old age? Or are you consuming junk food everyday that you can't even realistically see yourself being healthy past the age of 50?

As you are visualising these, I want you to write down any thoughts that passed through your head as you see these images. Are there any new priorities that you didn't know existed? Any shift in your bucket list?

Anything that jumped out to the front of the queue that you need to fix right this second? or to start doing right now?

If you are done I want you to open your eyes. How did that feel? Was it a surreal feeling to imagine yourself dying and looking back on your life, your teens, your 20s, your 30s. What were your biggest regrets and biggest accomplishments?

I want you to take this bucket list with you and take action on them. If you can prioritise them according to practicality, do it. If there are some easy tasks that you want to execute in next 6months, I want you to start them now. If your goal is to make some new friends that you can take to your golden years, I want you to start searching for them now so that you don't end up old and alone. Being lonely is one of the worst things that can happen to you, and I dont wish that on anyone. If you need to build up some friendships, dont waste time, because friendships takes time to nurture, and you don't want to end up in a situation that you don't have anyone to look for support, comfort, and simple companionship as you grow old.

I challenge each and everyone of you to live your life to the fullest, to live a life without regret, and that starts by taking action on the things that matters the most. It is not always about becoming a millionaire or a billionaire, because money can't buy everything. Money can't buy friends, it can't buy companionship, and it will not last. Build and create things that you can take with you right up to your death bed. And Remind yourself that life is short and not worth wasting.

Today we're going to talk about a topic that hopefully helps you become more aware of who you are as a person. And why do you exist right here and right now on this Earth. Because if we don't know who we are, if we don't understand ourselves, then how can we expect to other stand and relate to others? And why we even matter?

How many of you think that you can describe yourself accurately? If someone were to ask you exactly who you are, what would you say? Most of us would say we are Teachers, doctors, lawyers, etc. We would associate our lives with our profession.

But is that really what we are really all about?

Today I want to ask you not what you do, and not let your career define you, but rather what makes you feel truly alive and connected with the world? What is it about your profession that made you want to dedicated your life and time to it? Is there something about the job that makes you want to get up everyday and show up for the work, or is it merely to collect the paycheck at the end of the month?

I believe that that there is something in each and everyone of us that makes us who we are, and keeps us truly alive and full. For those that dedicate their lives to be Teachers, maybe they see themselves as an educator, a role model, a person who is in charge of helping a kid grow up, a nurturer, a parental figure. For Doctors, maybe they see themselves as healers, as someone who feels passionate about bringing life to someone. Whatever it may be, there is more to them than their careers.

For me, I see myself as a future caregiver, and to enrich the lives of my family members. That is something that I feel is one of my purpose in life. That I was born, not to provide for my family monetary per se, but to provide the care and support for them in their old age. That is one of my primary objectives. Otherwise, I see and understand myself as a person who loves to share knowledge with others, as I am doing right now. I love to help others in some way of form, either to inspire them, to lift their spirits, or to just be there for them when they need a crying shoulder. I love to help others fulfill their greatest potential, and it fills my heart with joy knowing that someone has benefitted from my advice. From what I have to say. And that what i have to say actually does hold some merit, some substance, and it is helping the lives of someone out there.. to help them make better decisions, and to help the, realise that life is truly wonderful. That is who i am.

Whenever I try to do something outside of that sphere, when what I do does not help someone in some way or another, I feel a sense of dread. I feel that what I do becomes misaligned with my calling, and I drag my feet each day to get those tasks done. That is something that I have realized about myself. And it might be happening to you too.

If u do not know exactly who you are and why you are here on this Earth, i highly encourage you to take the time to go on a self-discovery journey, however long it may take, to figure that out. Only when you know exactly who you are, can you start doing the work that aligns with ur purpose and calling. I don't meant this is in a religious way, but i believe that each and every one of us are here for a reason, whether it may to serve others, to help your fellow human beings, or to share your talents with the world, we should all be doing something with our lives that is at least close to that, if not exactly that.

So I challenge each and everyone of you to take this seriously because I believe you will be much happier for it. Start aligning your work with your purpose and you will find that life is truly worth living.

Chapter 3:
10 Habits That Will Make Your Life Better

All of us desire to have better lives. We hope that someday we will have progressive and substantive lives. We should be alive to the fact that a dream without concrete plans to realize it will remain just that – a dream on paper. Our habits cumulatively bring us closer to a better life. Here are ten habits that will make your life better:

1. Honesty

Success is founded on honest work. Honesty is the backbone of a better life. To succeed, you have to be honest with yourself and other people. Doing honest work and relating with people truthfully will establish you as reliable.

Honesty is rare and when people perceive you are reliable, they will entrust you with their resources and other factors of production

2. Continuously Learning New Things

We are in a constant state of learning. It is a continuous endless process that helps us become better daily. Even the most educated people have a new life concept to learn from other people. In learning, we unlearn myths, fallacies, and misconceptions. You can improve your life by learning a new skill that will aid you to face new challenges in life. Not everything is learned in a classroom, some lessons are acquired through experience. Purpose to learn throughout your life and your life will improve.

3. Accepting Correction

Nobody is perfect. Everybody has their flaws and the earlier you identify your weaknesses and work on them, the better things will get for you. Correction does not mean that you are incompetent but rather imperfect like everybody else.

Own up to your mistakes and do not be defensive when you are corrected. The first step towards improvement is accepting your wrongs and implementing the right suggestions.

4. Boldness To Make Tough Decisions

Sometimes you need to make landmark decisions in your life. It could be severing close ties with some people or being ruthless in abandoning old retrogressive habits. A better life is guaranteed if you make the right decisions. Fortune favors the bold. Better opportunities will come when you venture into new business spaces. Although the hesitancy in trying new things is real, evaluate the possible value arising from the bold step you will take.

5. Good Socializing Habits

Making friends fast is an important life skill. It is beneficial for you to easily blend in a given setting and make friends with strangers. When you are in a new space, get to know people because they can help you navigate unfamiliar territories. Good socializing habits will protect you from attacks when new people you meet profile you as unfriendly.

6. Quick Adaptability To The Environment

Do not seek preferential treatment whenever you are in a new environment. Adapt to the prevailing conditions and you will blend well with the local population.Moreover, you can focus on other important issues when you spend little time settling down. Quick adaptability will make you live peacefully wherever life takes you.

7. Creativity

Creativity can hardly be learned formally. It is mostly acquired through experience and personal zeal. Life is a cycle with many unique challenges. You cannot tackle every challenge in the same way.
Creativity will help you come up with new ways of approaching issues. Things will work out for you when you think out of the ordinary.

8. Building Bridges

It is important not to create enmity everywhere you go because you could be unknowingly shutting doors to future opportunities. Build bridges and not walls with people you meet because the future is uncertain. Life would be easier when you do not have many enemies to worry about. Your focus would be on more important matters.

9. Consulting

Nobody has a monopoly on ideas. Seeking advice is not a sign of weakness but an appreciation that you do not know everything. You have nothing to lose and instead stand to gain a lot from the advice you get. Instead of acting blindly, consult experienced people on issues you are naïve at. Consultation is an eye-opener to many things. You can thereafter make sober decisions.

10. Complying With Authority

Every place has rules that govern the place. Law brings order and streamlines issues where there is no clarity. Seek to fulfill what is required of you wherever you are by the existing authority. It is responsible for the creation of a conducive working environment. When you comply with set rules, you contribute to your success and that of others.

In conclusion, these ten habits will make your life better. They are the existing habits of successful people. We can be like them when we follow in their steps.

Chapter 4:

How To Have Proper Time Management

Managing time is one of the hardest things to do; our everyday routine revolves around time management. But what does it mean? Some people fail to understand the true meaning of time management. Time management can be defined as planning and controlling how much time to spend on specific activities. When a person knows how to manage his time, he faces less stress and efficiently completes more work in less time.

Everyone now wants to manage their time, the world is moving fast, so must we, but how to do that? The answer is relatively easy. You need to set your goals correctly. Setting your goals correctly would help you save time and so your brain wouldn't be messed up. The SMART method is the best method, where s stands for specific, M stands for measurable, A stands for attainable, R stands for relevant, and T stands for timely. If you set your goals by using the SMART method, you are bound to manage your time.

Now sometimes we all have so much work to do that we forget which one is more important, what you should do is to sit back for a minute, take out your to-do list and see which of your daily task is both important as well as urgent than that task should be your priority and you should do these tasks right away. Some tasks are important but not urgent, you can decide when to do these, but some are neither critical nor urgent you can leave them later to do. Prioritizing your tasks properly helps you manage time.

We all say that this generation is moving fast, but we also know that laziness is in the air. Being lazy is what messes up our routine. "Time is money" we all have heard this but hardly pay attention to this; wasting our time on one task is like ruining our whole plan for the day. You need to set a time limit for every task, depending on its difficulty level. When you have been assigned something to do, estimate the time it would take you to complete that task and set a limit. If you think you don't have enough time to complete the task, then seeking help from someone is not a bad option. But if you don't check the time, you may end up with incomplete work that will cause you a few problems.

Although work is essential, "All work and no play makes Jack a dull boy," this means that when a person is constantly working and burdens himself with the workload, he finds it hard to concentrate because his brain is all fried up. When you have a busy and packed schedule that includes many tasks, try to take small breaks between these tasks. Working constantly will make it hard for you to focus on your next task. You should take a break in the middle of these tasks, try grabbing a brief nap, or you can do something that will freshen up your brain like meditation, jogging, etc.

An organized person feels less messed up; for example, even if your wardrobe is messed up, you feel uncomfortable because this nagging sensation at the back of your head tells you that your closet needs to be organized. Similarly, try managing your calendar for more long-term time management. Try writing on a calendar about appointments, meetings, deadlines, so you don't forget what to do next. If there is something you need to do, then set a few days for that specific task. This method will help you remember more of your task and your plans.

Although time management is hard, it is not impossible. You just need to prioritise, take small breaks and sort out everything and you would be good to go.

Chapter 5:
7 Ways To Stop Overthinking And Relieve Stress

The way you respond to your thoughts can sometimes keep you in a cycle of <u>rumination</u>, or repetitive thinking. The next time you find yourself continuously running things over in your mind, take note of how it affects your mood. Do you feel irritated, nervous, or guilty? What's the primary emotion behind your thoughts? Having self-awareness is key to changing your mindset.

1. Find a distraction

Shut down overthinking by involving yourself in an activity you enjoy. This looks different for everyone, but ideas include:
- learning some new kitchen skills by tackling a new recipe
- going to your favorite workout class
- taking up a new hobby, such as painting
- volunteering with a local organization

2. Take a deep breath

You've heard it a million times, but that's because it works. The next time you find yourself tossing and turning over your thoughts, close your eyes and <u>breathe deeply</u>.

Try it

Here's a good starter exercise to help you unwind with your breath:

- Find a comfortable place to sit and relax your neck and shoulders.
- Place one hand over your heart and the other across your belly.
- Inhale and exhale through your nose, paying attention to how your chest and stomach move as you breathe.

Try doing this exercise three times a day for 5 minutes, or whenever you have racing thoughts.

3. Meditate

Developing a regular meditation practice is an evidence-backed way to help clear your mind of nervous chatter by turning your attention inward.

Look at the bigger picture

How will all the issues floating around in your mind affect you 5 or 10 years from now? Will anyone really care that you bought a fruit plate for the potluck instead of baking a pie from scratch?

Don't let minor issues turn into significant hurdles.

Do something nice for someone else

Trying to ease the load for someone else can help you put things in perspective. Think of ways you can be of service to someone going through a difficult time.

Does your friend who's in the middle of a divorce need a few hours of childcare? Can you pick up groceries for your neighbor who's been sick?

Realizing you have the power to make someone's day better can keep negative thoughts from taking over. It also gives you something productive to focus on instead of your never-ending stream of thoughts.

4. Recognize automatic negative thinking

Automated negative thoughts (ANTs) refer to knee-jerk negative thoughts, usually involving fear or anger, you sometimes have in reaction to a situation.

Tackling ANTs

You can identify and work through your ANTs by keeping a record of your thoughts and actively working to change them:

Use a notebook to track the situation giving you anxiety, your mood, and the first thought that comes to you automatically.

As you dig into details, evaluate why the situation is causing these negative thoughts.

Break down the emotions you're experiencing and try to identify what you're telling yourself about the situation.

Find an alternative to your original thought. For example, instead of jumping straight to, "This is going to be an epic failure," try something along the lines of, "I'm genuinely trying my best."

5. Acknowledge your successes

When you're in the midst of overthinking, stop and take out your notebook or your favorite note-taking app on your phone. Jot down five things that have gone right over the past week and your role in them.

These don't need to be huge accomplishments. Maybe you stuck to your coffee budget this week or cleaned out your car. When you look at it on paper or on-screen, you might be surprised at how these little things add up. If it feels helpful, refer back to this list when you find your thoughts spiralling.

6. Stay present

Not ready to commit to a meditation routine? There are plenty of other ways to ground yourself in the present moment.

Be here now

Here are a few ideas:

Unplug. Shut off your computer or phone for a designated amount of time each day, and spend that time on a single activity.

Eat mindfully. Treat yourself to one of your favorite meals. Try to find the joy in each bite, and really focus on how the food tastes, smells, and feels in your mouth.

Get outside. Take a walk outside, even if it's just a quick lap around the block. Take inventory of what you see along the way, noting any smells that waft by or sounds you hear.

7. Consider other viewpoints

Sometimes, quieting your thoughts requires stepping outside of your usual perspective. How you see the world is shaped by your life experiences, values, and assumptions. Imagining things from a different point of view can help you work through some of the noise

Chapter 6:
Discovering Your Strengths and Weaknesses

Today we're going to talk about a very simple yet important topic that hopefully brings about some self discovery about who you really are. By the end of this video i wish to help you find out what areas you are weak at so that maybe you could work on those, and what your strengths are so that you can play to them and lean into them more for greater results in your career and life in general.

We should all learn to accept our flaws as much as we embrace our strengths. And we have to remember that each of us are unique and we excel in different areas. Some of us are more artistic, some visionary, some analytical, some hardworking, some lazy, what matters is that we make these qualities work for us in our own special way.

Let's start by identifying your weaknesses. For those of you that have watched enough of my videos, you would know that i encourage all of you to take a pen to write things down. So lets go through this exercise real quick. Think of a few things that people have told you that you needed to work on, be it from your Teachers, your friends, your family, or whoever it may be.

How many of these weaknesses would you rate as significantly important that it would affect your life in a drastic way if you did not rectify it? I want you to put them at the top of your list. Next spend some time to reflect and look in the mirror. Be honest with yourself and identify the areas about yourself that you know needs some work.

Now I want you to take some time to identity your strengths. Repeat the process from above, what are the things people have told you about yourself that highlighted certain qualities about you? Whether that you're very outgoing, friendly, a great singer, a good team player, very diligent. I want you to write as many of these down as you can. No matter how big or small these strengths are, I want you to write down as many as you can.

Now I want you to also place your 3 biggest strengths at the top of the list. As I believe these are the qualities that best represent who you are as a person.

Now that you've got these 2 lists. I want you to compare them. Which list is longer? the one with strengths or weaknesses? If you have more weaknesses, that's okay, it just means that there is more room for improvement. If you have more strengths, thats good.

What we are going to do with this list now is to now make it a mission to improve our weaknesses and play heavily into our strengths for the foreseeable future. You see, our strengths are strengths for a reason, we are simply naturally good at it. Whether it be through genetics, or our personalities, or the way we have been influenced by the world. We should all try to showcase our strengths as much as we can. It is hard for me to say exactly what that is, but I believe that you will know how you maximise the use of your talent. Whether it be serving others, performing for others, or even doing specific focused tasks. Simply do more of it. Put yourself in more situations where you can practice these strengths. And keep building on it. It will take little effort but yield tremendous results.

As for your weaknesses, I want you to spend some time on the top 3 that you have listed so far. As these could be the areas that have been holding you back the most. Making improvements in these areas could be the breakthrough that you need to become a much better person and could see you achieving a greater level success than if you had just left them alone.

I challenge each and everyone of you to continually play to your strengths, sharpening them until they are sharp as a knife, while working on smoothening the rough edges of your weaknesses. So that they may balance out your best qualities.

Chapter 7:

How Much Is Your Time Really Worth?

What is the biggest mistake we make in life? Perhaps Buddha's most suitable answer was given by "The biggest mistake is you think you have time." While our time in this world is free, it's also priceless. We can neither own it nor keep it, but we can use it and spend it. And once it's all lost, it's inevitable that we will never get it back.

"Your time is limited, so don't waste it living someone else's life." - Steve Jobs. Our time is limited in this world is both good and bad news. The bad news is that time flies and never returns, but the good news is that we're the pilot. The average person lives 78 years on this planet. We spend almost one-third of our lives sleeping; that's approximately 28.3 years from our lives. And still, 30% of us struggle to sleep well. We spend almost 10.5 years of our life working, but over 50% of us want to leave our current jobs. Time is a valuable asset, even more so than money. We can get more money, but we can never get more time.

After all of the years we spend doing chores, shopping, grooming, eating, drinking, TV, and social media, time leaves us with only nine years. Now the question arises, how will we spend that time? Just like we would never waste our money on something gratuitous, why do we waste our time on it? We might think that people are wasting our time when we are the ones permitting them to do that in reality. We sometimes end up losing our most beloved people because we don't value their time. Some of us don't recognize their importance until they're gone.

Every day, from the moment we wake up till the moment we get back to sleep, two voices are battling inside our heads; one wants to uplift us and one that holds us back. And which one will win? The one that we listen to the most. The one that we feed us the most. The one that we amplify. Similarly, it's up to us and our choice how we use that time in our hands. William Shakespeare once said, "Time is prolonged for those who want, very fast for those who are scared, very long for those who are sad, and very short for those who celebrate, but for those who love, time is eternal." We should make the most out of our time and learn its value by carefully analyzing what life teaches us about it.

Chapter 8:
The Keys To Happiness

If I ask you "what is happiness?", then what would your answer be? It's probably difficult to come up with a simple answer. Yet, here you are, looking for a key to happiness and how to lead a fulfilling life.

The truth is that a universal key to happiness is a myth.

That doesn't mean that you should stop looking for yours right now, it only means that you need to be careful when reading articles about "a key to happiness". The universal key to happiness is non-existent because happiness is one of the most difficult things in life to define.

Now, let's go back to that difficult question: "what is happiness?"

Have you thought about it already? Let me give you an example of how hard it is to define happiness.

Right now, I'm drinking a cup of coffee while writing the outline of this article about how to define happiness. Am I happy right now? Yes, I'm feeling pretty happy:

- I've got nothing to worry about.
- All my basic needs are met.
- The weather is nice.
- I'm going outside in a couple of minutes to go for a walk.

These things are all making me feel pretty happy right now.

By that logic, let's define my happiness as follows:

"Happiness is when I'm in a worry-free state, the weather is nice, everybody I know is alright and I can enjoy a hot cup of coffee."

Voila. There it is. My definition of happiness.

The keys to my happiness are obvious now, and I know enough in order to lead the happiest life I can. I just need to focus on the things I listed above.

Wait a second... If it were this simple, then why have I ever been unhappy?

You might have guessed it already, but I made a very simple error. I assumed that what makes me happy today will make me happy for the rest of my life. And that's just wrong.

Happiness is something that not only changes from person to person, but it's also constantly evolving from day to day.

Your definition of happiness changes over time. This is why happiness is such a difficult concept, and why there's not a single "key to happiness". Whoever tells you otherwise is likely not aware that people change, and that people don't always share the same values, goals, and purposes.

For a minute, I want you to do consider your own happiness. I want you to think back of last week, and consider what things you did that had a positive effect on your happiness.

What things had a significant influence on your mood? What comes to your mind?

Was it spending time with your friends? Was it a great movie you watched? Did you attend an exciting sports event? Or did you enjoy sipping hot coffee on a sunny Wednesday morning? It could obviously be just about anything! The most important thing to remember when trying to define your keys to a happy and fulfilling life is simple:

There is no universal key that leads to your happiness. That's because your happiness is unique in each and every single way

Chapter 9:
5 Ways To Deal with Personal Feelings of Inferiority

Have you at some point felt that you are inferior to others? That's normal. All of us, at some point in our lives, have felt the same. Growing up, we saw other kids who performed better than us in the class. Kids who played sports well. Kids who were loved by all. We got jealous. We felt inferior to them. We constantly compared ourselves to them.

Almost everyone has experienced that in their childhood. But do you still feel the same about others? Do you constantly analyze situations and people around you? Do you feel worthless? Then you probably have an inferiority complex. But the good news is you can get over this inferiority complex. We are going to list some of the things that will help you in doing that.

1. **Build self-confidence**

Treat yourself better. Act confident. Do what you love. Embrace yourself. Is there anything in your body that you don't feel confident about? Maybe your smile, your nose, or your hair? The trick here is to either accept yourself the way you are or do something about it. If you have curly hair, get your hair straightener. Do whatever makes you feel better about yourself.

2. Surround yourself with people who uplift you

It's important to realize that your inferiority complex might be linked to the people around you. It might be your relatives, your friends at college, your siblings, or your colleagues. Analyze your interactions with them.

Once you can identify people who try to pull you down, do not reciprocate your feelings, or are not very encouraging, start distancing yourself from them. Look for positive people, who uplift you, and who bring out the better version of yourself. Take efforts to develop a relationship with them.

3. Stop worrying about what other people think.

One major cause of inferiority complexes is constantly thinking about what others are thinking about us. We seek validation from them for every action of ours. Sometimes we are thinking about their actions, while sometimes, we imagine what they think.

4. Stop worrying about what other people think.

One major cause of inferiority complexes is constantly thinking about what others are thinking about us. We seek validation from them for every action of ours. Sometimes we are thinking about their actions, while sometimes, we are imagining what they think.

Disassociate yourself from their judgments. It's ultimately your opinion about yourself that matters. When we feel good about ourselves, others feel good about ourselves.

5. Do not be harsh on yourself.

There is no need to be harsh on yourself. Practice self-care. Love yourself. Be kind to yourself. Do not over-analyze situations. Do not expect yourself to change overnight. Give yourself time to heal.

Chapter 10:
Happy People Stay Present

"Realize deeply that the present moment is all you ever have."

According to a study, 50% of the time, we are not fully present in the moment. We are either thinking about the past or worrying about the future. These things lead to frustration, anxiety, and pain in our daily life. Each morning as soon as we wake up, we start seeking distractions. As we wake up with a clear mind, we should be grateful for a new day that we got; instead, we start looking for our phone, start going through interwebs and rush into our days. So now we are going to help you and list some of the things that will help you stay present.

Stop Being a Slave to Your Mind: For the next four days, let's do an exercise where you pay attention to your thoughts and see what crosses your mind. You. You will soon realize that majority of the thoughts that you have are destructive. There will be very little time to think about the present, and the majority of your thoughts would be about the past or the future. So, whenever this happens and you find yourself wandering consciously, try to bring yourself back to the present. Also, you need to remind yourself that multi-tasking is a myth and focus on one thing only.

Tap into Your Senses: If you mindfully tap into your senses, you will realize that it is a fantastic way of bringing more awareness into your day. Because our eyes are wide open all day, we can see, but we forget to tap into other senses such as taste, touch, or smell. But if you use these, you can feel more present and calm down if you are in a stressful situation. You might not realize this, but our senses play a huge role in manifesting our reality. For example, everything we are hearing we are touching will regularly turn into our reality. That is why we can use the power our senses have and feel more calm and present.

Listen Closely: Everyone loves to talk, but only a few people like to listen. People love to share their dreams, what they have accomplished and what they desire, and still, nobody seems to be listening closely.

"When you talk, you are only repeating what you already know. But if you listen, you may learn something new."

When you listen carefully, you will be able to charm people and at the same time learn new things and be present. Because you will be focusing on what they are saying, you will focus on the current moment. This way, you will also be able to silence your thoughts about the past and future because you will be consciously listening and focusing on what they are saying. This will also benefit your relationship in the long run because when you need an ear to listen to your problems, they will be there for you. This is a win-win situation for you, and you will improve your relationship while practising being more present.

Chapter 11:
Productivity Mistake: Being in Motion Vs. Taking Action

There is a common mistake that often happens to smart people — in many cases, without you even realizing it. The mistake has to do with the difference between being in motion and taking action. They sound similar, but they're not the same.

Motion vs. Action

When you're in motion, you're planning and strategizing, and learning. Those are all good things, but they don't produce a result. Action, on the other hand, is the type of behavior that will deliver an outcome. Here are some examples...

- If I outline 20 ideas for articles I want to write, that's motion. If I write and publish an article, that's action.

- If I email ten new leads for my business and start conversations with them, that's motion. If they buy something and turn into a customer, that's action.

- If I search for a better diet plan and read a few books on the topic, that's motion. If I eat a healthy meal, that's action.

Sometimes motion is useful, but it will never produce an outcome by itself. It doesn't matter how many times you go talk to the personal trainer. That motion will never get you in shape. Only the action of working out will get the result you're looking to achieve.

Why Smart People Find Themselves in Motion

If the motion doesn't lead to results, why do we do it? Sometimes we do it because we need to plan or learn more. But more often than not, we do it because motion allows us to feel like we're making progress without running the risk of failure. Most of us are experts at avoiding criticism. It doesn't feel good to fail or be judged publicly, so we tend to avoid situations where that might happen. And that's the biggest reason why you slip into motion rather than taking action: you want to delay failure.

Yes, I'd like to get in shape. But I don't want to look stupid in the gym, so I'll just talk to the trainer about their rates instead.

Yes, I'd like to land more clients for my business. But, if I ask for the sale, I might get turned down. So maybe I should just email ten potential clients instead.

It's easy to be in motion and convince yourself that you're still making progress. Motion makes you feel like you're getting things done. But really, you're just preparing to get something done. When preparation becomes a form of procrastination, you need to change something. You don't want to merely be planning. You want to be practicing.

The motion will never produce a final result. Action will. When you're in motion, you're planning and strategizing, and learning. Those are all good things, but they don't produce a result. Today take five minutes out and ask yourself, Are you doing something? Or are you just preparing to do it? Are you in motion? Or are you taking action?

Chapter 12:
Happy People Don't Sweat the Small Stuff.

Stress follows a peculiar principle: when life hits us with big crises—the death of a loved one or a job loss—we somehow find the inner strength to endure these upheavals in due course. It's the little things that drive us insane day after day—traffic congestion, awful service at a restaurant, an overbearing coworker taking credit for your work, meddling in-laws, for example.

It's all too easy to get caught up in the many irritations of life. We overdramatize and overreact to life's myriad tribulations. Under the direct influence of anguish, our minds are bewildered, and we feel disoriented. This creates stress, which makes the problems more difficult to deal with.

The central thesis of psychotherapist Richard Carlson's bestselling ***Doesn't Sweat The Small Stuff… And It's All Small Stuff*** (1997) is this: to deal with angst or anger, we need not some upbeat self-help prescriptions for changing ourselves, but simply a measure of perspective.

Perspective helps us understand that there's an art to understand what we should let go of and what we should concern ourselves with. It is important to focus our efforts on the important stuff and not waste time on insignificant and incidental things.

I've previously written about my favorite [5-5-5 technique](#) for gaining perspective and guarding myself against [anger erupting](#): I remove myself from the offending environment and contemplate if whatever I'm getting worked up over is of importance. I ask myself, "Will this matter in 5 days? Will this matter in 5 months? Will this matter in 5 years?"

Carlson stresses that there's always a vantage point from which even the biggest stressor can be effectively dealt with. The challenge is to keep making that shift in perspective. When we achieve that ["wise-person-in-me" perspective](#), our problems seem more controllable and our lives more peaceful.

Carlson's prescriptions aren't uncommon—we can learn to be more patient, compassionate, generous, grateful, and kind, all of which will improve the way we feel about ourselves and how other people feel when they are around us.

Some of Carlson's 100 recommendations are trite and banal—for example, "make peace with imperfection," "think of your problems as potential teachers," "remember that when you die, your 'in-basket' won't be empty," and "do one thing at a time." Others are more informative:

- Let others have the glory
- Let others be "right" most of the time
- Become aware of your moods, and don't allow yourself to be fooled by the low ones
- Look beyond behavior
- Every day, tell at least one person something you like, admire, or appreciate about them.
- Argue for your limitations, and they're yours
- Resist the urge to criticize
- Read articles and books with entirely different points of view from your own and try to learn something.

Chapter 13:
Motivation With Good Feelings

Ever wonder what goes on in your mind when you feel depressed isn't always the reaction to the things that happen to you? What you go through when you feel down is the chemistry of your brain that you yourself allow being created in the first place.

You don't feel weak just because your heart feels so heavy. You feel weak because you have filled your heart with all these feelings that don't let you do something useful.

Feelings are not your enemy till you choose the wrong ones. In fact, Feelings and emotions can be the strongest weapon to have in your arsenal.

People say, "You are a man, so act like one. Men don't cry, they act strong and brave"

You must make yourself strong enough to overcome any feelings of failure or fear. Any thought that makes you go aloof and dims that light of creativity and confidence. It's OK to feel sad and cry for some time, but it's not OK to feel weak for even a second.

Your consciousness dictates your feelings. Your senses help you to process a moment and in turn help you translate them into feelings that go both ways. This process has been going on from the day you were born and will continue till your last day.

You enter your consciousness as soon as you open your eyes to greet the day. It is at this moment when your creativity is at its peak. What you need now is just a set of useful thoughts and emotions that steer your whole day into a worthwhile one.

Don't spend your day regretting and repressing things you did or someone else did to you. You don't need these feelings right now. Because you successfully passed those tests of life and are alive still to be grateful for what you have right now.

There are a billion things in life to be thankful for and a billion more to be sad for. But you cannot live a happy fulfilling life if you focus on the later ones.

Life is too short to be sad and to be weak. When you start your day, don't worry about what needs to be done. But think about who you need to be to get those things done.

Don't let actions and outcomes drive you. Be the sailor of yourself to decide what outcomes you want.

Believe me, the feeling of gratitude is the biggest motivator. Self gratitude should be the level of appraisal to expect. Nothing should matter after your own opinions about yourself.

If you let other people's opinions affect your feelings, you are the weakest person out there. And failure is your destination.

Visualization of a better life can help you feel and hope better. It would help you to grow stronger and faster but remember; The day you lose control of your emotions, feelings, and your temper, your imagination will only lead you to a downward spiral.

Chapter 14:
7 Ways To Attract Happiness

We have seen a lot of people defining success as to their best of knowledge. While happiness is subjective from person to person, there's a law of attraction that remains constant for everyone in the world. It states that you will indirectly start to attract all the good things in life when you become happier. This is why happy people often have good lives where everything just somehow tends to work for them. Happiness not only feels good but can also make our manifestation attempts twice as effective. We shouldn't measure our happiness from external factors but instead, as cliche as it may sound, we should know that true happiness comes from the inside.

Here are some ways for you to attract happiness:

1. **Make a choice to be happy:**

When you choose to be as happy as you can in every moment of your life, your subconscious mind will start acknowledging your decision, and it will begin to find ways to bring more joy into your life. When you work towards your decision of being happy, the universe also plays its part and makes sure it attracts more situations in your life that you can be pleased about. The positive vibrations that you will give out will find their way back to you. You don't have to make the decision of being happy right away, as some of you might be going through a tough time. Sit, relax, and take some time to reflect on yourself first and then make a choice whenever you're ready.

2. Define What Happiness Means To You

We have also found ourselves asking this question a million times, "what exactly is happiness?" Some people would attach the idea of happiness with materialistic things such as a big house, expensive cars, branded clothes and shoes, designer bags, the latest technologies, and so forth. While for some, happiness is merely spending time with family and friends, doing the things that they love, and finding inner peace and calm.

3. React Positively under all situations:

We could experience a thousand good things but a million bad ones in our everyday lives. And sometimes, it could be complicated for us to encounter any kind of happiness given the circumstances. Although these circumstances cannot be in our control, how we react to them is always in our hands. As our favorite Professor Dumbledore once said, "Happiness can be found even in the darkest of times if only one remembers to turn on the light." Similarly, we should always try to find that silver lining at the end of the dark tunnel, always seek some positivity in every situation. But we are only humans. Don't try to enforce positivity on yourself if you don't feel like it. It's okay to address all our emotions equally till you be yourself again.

4. Do not procrastinate:

You might find it a bit weird, but procrastination does snatch your happiness away. No matter how much things are going well in your life, you would always find a loophole, a reason to be unhappy and dissatisfy with yourself a well as your life. Procrastination makes you believe that you are not living up to your fullest potential. You will get this nagging feeling that will eventually morph into negative emotions that would nearly eat you. So, try to avoid procrastination as much as possible and start doing the things that actually matter.

5. **Stay present:**

The key to becoming more focused, more at peace, more effective in manifesting, and eventually, much happier is to just live in the moment. Whatever you're doing in the present, try to be completely aware and focused on it. It will help you avoid all the negative feelings you have conjured up about the past and future. Try to stay present as much as you can; over time, it will become a habit, and you will develop the capability to face it all. This will definitely help you attract more happiness into your life.

6. **Do not compare yourself:**

As Theodore Rosevelt once said, "Comparison is the thief of joy." Whenever we compare ourselves to others, we tend to become ungrateful and strip ourselves of the ability to appreciate the good and abundance in our lives. We start to magnify the good in other people's lives and the bad that is in our own. We must understand that everyone is going through their own pace, and they all are secretly struggling with one thing or the other.

7. Don't try too hard:

Happiness demands patience. It is better to get into it gradually rather than being overeager. Many people take the law of attraction and being positive a little too far and start obsessing over it. They tend to panic if they get negative thoughts or are unable to attract the things they want. Don't get frustrated if things don't work out your way, and don't give up on the idea of happiness if you feel distressed. Try to prioritize your happiness and give others a reason to be happy too. Make yours as well as other's lives easy.

Conclusion:

Not many people know that, but being happy is actually the foundation towards attracting all your dreams and goals. When you adopt the habit of becoming truly happy every day, everything good will naturally follow you. Over time, happiness can even become your default state. Try your best to follow the guidelines above, and I guarantee that you will start feeling happier immediately.

Chapter 15:
Trust The Process

Today we're going to talk about the power of having faith that things will work out for you even though you can't see the end in sight just yet. And why you need to simply trust in the process in all the things that you do.

Fear is something that we all have. We fear that if we quit our jobs to pursue our passions, that we may not be able to feed ourselves if our dreams do not work out. We fear that if we embark on a new business venture, that it might fail and we would have incurred financial and professional setbacks.

All this is borne out of the fear of the unknown. The truth is that we really do not know what can or will happen. We may try to imagine in our heads as much as we can, but we can never really know until we try and experienced it for ourselves.

The only way to overcome the fear of the unknown is to take small steps, one day at a time. We will, to the best of our ability, execute the plan that we have set for ourselves. And the rest we leave it up to the confidence that our actions will lead to results.

If problems arise, we deal with it there and then. We put out fires, we implement updated strategies, and we keep going. We keep going until we have exhausted all avenues. Until there is no more roads for us to travel, no more paths for us to create. That is the best thing that we can do.

If we constantly focus on the fear, we will never go anywhere. If we constantly worry about the future, we will never be happy with the present. If we dwell on our past failures, we will be a victim of our own shortcomings. We will not grow, we will not learn, we will not get better.

I challenge each and every one of you today to make the best out of every situation that you will face. Grab fear by the horns and toss them aside as if it were nothing. I believe in you and all that you can achieve.

Chapter 16:
Stop Being a Slave To Old Beliefs

Life has a beginning for everyone. Everyone has a different life. Everyone has a different belief. Everyone has different brains and different observations. You are that everyone. You are different in every aspect possible except the fact that you are only human life to a billion others.

We humans, as a species have lived history through a certain set of rules. Modern and civilized cultures live with some social decorum and follow some societal beliefs and rituals. But who imposed these laws on us?

Who made these rituals so important for everyone, as if we cannot survive without them? There is no justification for most of these beliefs that are still being practiced to date.

Humans have also the same ways of adapting to thins like other animals. They tend to repeat things to perfect or learn them.

We have practiced so many pointless beliefs and conditions for so long that we are unwilling and unable to even try to think aside them.

We are so scared to look around these beliefs and shake things up a bit to create newer and better outcomes for us and others. But we still feel liable and a slave to this tendency to follow whatever is being imposed on us. No!

You are a free soul. You were born a free soul. You were given a unique mind and you should act like you still have one. You can think of bigger and better ways to make your life easier and more meaningful.

Look at a bird. They start taking lessons from other birds, but when they are finally in the air for the first time, they are now free to do anything they can ever wish to do.

You are also a free bird. You have everything you want to create new beliefs of your own where you don't have to justify or answer to anyone because now you have a person to fall back on. And that person is You!

What if you started a cult today, and someone came and asked you to justify it. Do you think you owe that person an answer? I don't think so!

Because you are a free individual who can anything he or she wants, only if it doesn't hurt anyone else around you.

You started your life alone and you will die alone. So why not live it alone too. I am not saying to give up on all relations. But you should make up your own beliefs if you are not OK with the previous ones.

Don't argue! You cannot force your opinion on anyone else, just like you are not obligated to follow anyone else's.

So from this day in your life. Make a vow to yourself, that you will take every day of your life as if it were a new life and you will discover newer things this time. This will help you find a newer purpose and will eventually create a new ambition for others to follow.

Chapter 17:
Deal With Your Fears Now

Fear is a strange thing.

Most of our fears are phantoms that never actually appear or become real,

Yet it holds such power over us that it stops us from making steps forward in our lives.

It is important to deal with fear as it not only holds you back but also keeps you caged in irrational limitations.

Your life is formed by what you think.

It is important not to dwell or worry about anything negative.

Don't sweat the small stuff, and it's all small stuff (Richard Carlson).

It's a good attitude to have when avoiding fear.

Fear can be used as a motivator for yourself.

If you're in your 30s, you will be in your 80s in 50 years, then it will be too late.

And that doesn't mean you will even have 50 years. Anything could happen.

But let's say you do, that's 50 years to make it and enjoy it.

But to enjoy it while you are still likely to be healthy, you have a maximum of 15 years to make it - minus sleep and living you are down to 3 years.

If however you are in your 40s, you better get a move on quickly.

Does that fear not dwarf any possible fears you may have about taking action now?

Dealing with other fears becomes easy when the ticking clock is staring you in the face.

Most other fears are often irrational.

We are only born with two fears, the fear of falling and the fear of load noises.

The rest have been forced on us by environment or made up in our own minds.

The biggest percentage of fear never actually happens.

To overcome fear we must stare it in the face and walk through it knowing our success is at the other side.

Fear is a dream killer and often stops people from even trying.

Whenever you feel fear and think of quitting, imagine behind you is the ultimate fear of the clock ticking away your life.

If you stop you lose and the clock is a bigger monster than any fear.

If you let anything stop you the clock will catch you.

So stop letting these small phantoms prevent you from living,

They are stealing your seconds, minutes, hours , days and weeks.

If you carry on being scared, they will take your months, years and decades.

Before you know it they have stolen your life.

You are stronger than fear but you must display true strength that fear will be scared.
It will retreat from your path forever if you move in force towards it because fear is fear and by definition is scared.

We as humans are the scariest monsters on planet Earth.
So we should have nothing to fear
Fear tries to stop us from doing our life's work and that is unacceptable.
We must view life's fears as the imposters they are, mere illusions in our mind trying to control us.

We are in control here.
We have the free will to do it anyway despite fear.
Take control and fear will wither and disappear as if it was never here.
The control was always yours you just let fear steer you off your path.

Fear of failure, fear of success, fear of what people will think.
All irrational illusions.
All that matters is what you believe.
If your belief and faith in yourself is strong , fear will be no match for your will.

Les Brown describes fear as false evidence appearing real.
I've never seen a description so accurate.

Whenever fear rears its ugly head, just say to yourself this is false evidence appearing real.

Overcoming fear takes courage and strength in one's self.

We must develop more persistence than the resistance we will face when pursuing our dreams.

If we do not develop a thick skin and unwavering persistence we will be beaten by fear, loss and pain.

Our why must be so important that these imposters become small in comparison.

Because after all the life we want to live does dwarf any fears or set back that might be on the path.

Fear is insignificant.

Fear is just one thing of many we must beat into the ground to prove our worth.

Just another test that we must pass to gain our success.

Because success isn't your right,

You must fight

With all your grit and might

Make it through the night and shine your massive light on the world.

And show everyone you are a star.

Chapter 18:
Bounce Back From Failure

Failure is a big word. It is a negative word most say. It is cursed in most cases. It is frowned upon when it is on your plate. But why?

Sure, it certainly doesn't feel good when you encounter failure. We can't even forgive ourselves for failing at a simple card game. We get impatient, we get hopeless and ultimately we get depressed on even the smallest of failure we go through in everyday life.

Why is it that way? Why can't we try to change a failure into something better? Why can't we just leave that failure right there and not try to make a big deal out of each and every small little setback?

These questions have a very deep meaning and a very important place in everyone's life.

Let's start with the simplest step to make it easy for yourself to deal with a certain failure. Whenever you fail at anything, just pause for a second and talk to yourself.

Rewind what you just went through. Talk to yourself through the present circumstances. Think about what you could have done to improve at what you just did. Think about what you could have done to prevent whatever tragic incident you went through. Or what you could have done to do better at what you felt like failing at.

These questions will immediately sketch a scenario in front of your eyes. A scenario where you can actually see yourself flourishing and doing your best against all odds.

Whatever happened to you, I am sure you didn't deserve it. But so what if you

Lost some money or a loved one or your pet? Ask yourself this, is it the end of the world? Have you stopped breathing? Have you no reason left to keep living?

You had, you have, and you will always have a new thing, a new person a new place to start with. Life has endless possibilities for you to find. But you just have to bounce back from whatever setback you think you cannot get out of.

Take for example the biggest tech billionaires in the world. I am giving this example because people tend to relate more to these examples these days. Elon Musk started his carrier with a small office with his brother and they both lived in the same office for a whole year. They couldn't even afford a small place for themselves to rent.

There was a time when Elon had to decide to split his last set of investments between two companies. If he had invested in one, the other would have gone down for sure, just to give a chance to the other company to maybe become their one big hit. Guess what, he ended up keeping them both because he invested in both.

Why did he succeed? Was it because he wasn't afraid? No!

He succeeded because he had Faith after all the failures he had faced. He knew that if he kept trying against all odds and even the obvious risks, he will ultimately succeed at something for what he worked so hard for all this time!

Chapter 19:
How To Stop Procrastinating

Procrastination; perhaps the most used word of our generation. Procrastination can range from a minor issue that hurts your productivity or a significant issue that's preventing you from achieving your goals. You feel powerless, and you feel hopeless; you feel de-motivated, De-strategized, even guilty and ashamed, but all in vain.

Let me in all of you on a secret of life, the need to avoid pain and the desire to gain pleasure. That is what we consider the two driving forces of life. Repeat this mantra till it gets in the back of your head. And if you don't take control over these two forces, they'll take control over you and your entire life. The need to avoid pain is what gets us into procrastinating. We aren't willing to step out of our comfort zone, be uncomfortable, fear the pain of spending our energies, fear failure, embarrassment, and rejection. We don't simply procrastinate because there's no other choice; we procrastinate because whatever it is, we don't consider it essential to us. It's not that something meaningful for us or urgent to us, and when something doesn't feel binding to us, we tend to put it off. We link to link a lot of pain to not taking action. But what if we reversed the roles? What if we start to connect not taking action to be more painful than taking action. We have to change our perspective.

See that the long-term losses of not taking action are 1000x more painful than the short-term losses of taking those actions.

Stop focusing on the short-term pain of spending your time, energy, and emotions on the tasks at hand. START focusing on the long-term pain that comes when you'll realize you're not even close to the goals you were meant to achieve.

Stop your desire to gain pleasure from the unnecessary and unimportant stuff. You would rather skip your workout to watch a movie instead. You're focusing on the pleasure, the meaningless short-term craving that'll do you no good. Imagine the pleasure we'd gain if we actually did that workout. Stop making excuses for procrastinating. Start owning up to yourself, your tasks, your goals. Set a purpose in your life and start working tirelessly towards it. Take breaks but don't lose your focus!

If you're in school and you're not getting the grades that you want, and still you're not doing anything about it, then maybe it's not a priority for you. But how do we make it meaningful? How do we make it purposeful? You need to find that motivation to get yourself going. And I promise you once you find that purpose, you'll get up early in the morning, and you'll start working to make your dreams come true.

Don't just talk about it, be about it! You were willing to graduate this year, you were willing to go to the gym and change your physique, you were willing to write that book, but what happened? You didn't make them a priority, and you eventually got tired of talking. Take a deep breath and allow yourself to make the last excuse there is that's stopping you from whatever it is that you're supposed to do. I don't have enough money; I don't write well, I don't sing well, I don't have enough knowledge, that's it. That's the last excuse you're going to make and get it over with. Aren't you tired of feeling defeated? Aren't you tired of getting beat? Aren't you tired of saying "I'll get it done soon" over and over again? To all the procrastinators, YOU. STILL. HAVE. PLENTY. OF. TIME. Don't quit, don't give up, don't just lay there doing nothing; you can make it happen. But not with that procrastinating. Set up a goal, tear it into manageable pieces, stop talking about the things you were going to do, and start doing them for real!

It's not too late for anything. There might be some signs that'll show you that you need to rest. Take them. Take the time you need to get back on track. But don't give up on the immediate gratification. Don't listen to that little voice in your head. Get out of bed, lift those weights, start working on that project, climb that mountain. You're the only person that's stopping you from achieving your goals, your dreams. With long-term success, either you're going to kick the hell out of life, or life's going to kick the hell out of you; whichever of that happens the most will become your reality. We're the master of our fates, the ambassador of our ambitions; why waste our time and lives away into doing something that won't even matter to us in a few years? Why not work towards something that will touch people, inspire them, give them hope.

I'll do it in the next hour, I'll do it the next day, I'll do it the next week, and before you know, you're dragging it to the next month or even next year. And that's the pain of life punching you in the face. The regrets of missing opportunities will eventually catch up to you. Every day you get a chance to either make the most out of life or sit on the sidelines taking the crumbles which people are leaving behind. Take what you want or settle for what's left! That's your choice.

You have to push yourself long past the point of boredom. Boredom is your worst enemy. It kills more people in the pursuit of success than anything or anyone will ever destroy. Your life just doesn't stop accidentally. It's a series of actions that you either initiate or don't initiate. Some people have already made their big decisions today, after waking up. While some, they're still dwelling on the things that don't matter. They're afraid of self-evaluation, thus wasting their time. So focus on yourself, focus on what you're doing with your time, have clarity on what you're trying to achieve. Build into what you're trying to accomplish. Between where you are and where you want to go, there's a skill set that you have to master. There's a gap that's asking for your hard work. So pay the price for what you want to become.

Chapter 20:

Stop Wasting Time on the Details and Commit to the Fundamentals

Time runs on a treadmill that has no apparent switch. We have a timeline on this planet and it will come to an end sooner or later. It would be sooner than we think, that is for sure!

But what we put in, to live what time we have to make it matter for if it were our last second, is a concept I'll try to endorse here.

You see, we all live our lives as if no one is more sincere and dedicated than we are. We put in all the hours and we put in all the energy but we can't guarantee anything, can we?

It is never about how hardworking you are. It is never about the rules and the intricacies of things we follow. It is never about the hours we put in, but what we put into the hours!

This is not as simple as it may sound. We, humans, have a common flaw as an intelligent species. It is an adherent flaw in our upbringing and the norms that we follow.

We don't know what is more important, is it the plane or the pilot? We have what we call an instinctive nature that draws us to conclusions and things that will influence us to ultimately find our purpose, but in that process of finding one, we lose focus of what we have at hand right now!

We are working straight hours for things that have secondary importance in our lives and sometimes can be discouraging. We are working so hard on things that have least to no contribution to our happiness and success but we are still going on around them foolishly.

Not everything is meant to be done and not everything is meant to bring meaning to the spice of life. But we still do it because we are naive and shallow.

We need to learn what are the fundamentals of living a successful life.

You don't have a single aspect of your life to take care of. You can't dedicate the majority of your time and attention to fixing only one thing when there are a lot more and lot better things to take care of.

You don't need to avoid the bigger and bolder realities just because you are afraid you might fail and fall. You surely can and you surely will. You only have to keep trying and you will eventually set things straight.

Set your priorities in the right direction. You don't need a fancy logo for your business if you haven't had a single paying customer yet. You can't have a better grade if you haven't done any of the term work. You can't expect to be paid a full wager if you have dozens of chores still pending for the next day.

The details are useless if you haven't had the fundamentals done yet. The final formula has no meaning if you had the basic equation wrong. So follow the process and the process will lead you to the final viewpoint!

Chapter 21:
16 Steps To Stop Feeling Like Shit

We all have days where we feel like absolute crap and don't even feel like talking to anyone. There are some small steps that can help you feel better even if its just for a while.

1. Get a drink of water

You could be dehydrated! Your body needs water. Not juice, soda, or alcohol — get a tall glass of water and make yourself drink all of it.

2. Make your bed

When you have a lot to do and it feels overwhelming, making your bed can be the first step in getting your life on track. It will also (hopefully) discourage you from getting back into it.

3. Take a shower

Life feels different when you're clean! And it can give you a burst of energy if you're feeling lethargic. Wash your hair and give yourself a head massage.

4. Have a snack — not junk food!

Did you eat enough today? It's super tempting to eat junk food when you feel like crap. If you don't feel like making a whole meal, maybe eat just a piece of fruit; something you can burn throughout the day and not in a burst of five minutes.

5. Take a walk.

You might need some fresh air and not even know it. Give your body some natural light, breathe some different air, move your legs a little, even if it's for just five minutes. Allow yourself to think some different thoughts.

6. Change your clothes

Even if you aren't going to leave the house today, put on real clothes. Or, if you've been wearing the same uncomfortable clothes all day and feel restless, change into your sleepy clothes and slippers and relax.

7. Change your environment

Staring at the same four walls day after day can be drudging. Can you work from a cafe, a library, or a friend's house? If you can add going somewhere to the list of things you did today, you may feel more accomplished.

8. Talk to someone, not on the internet — it can be about anything

If you don't feel like talking through your troubles, that's OK. Visit a friend, talk to them about a movie you saw. Call your mom and see how she's doing.

9. Dance to an upbeat guilty pleasure song

NOT ELLIOT SMITH! Pick something high energy and bump it. Dance like a rock star for one song to get your blood pumping again.

10. Get some exercise

Do some cardio, work up a sweat. If you don't have the time for a whole workout, look up a sun salutation on YouTube and stretch for as long as you have time. Do some push-ups or sit-ups at your desk.

11. Accomplish something — even if it's something tiny

Do you need to grab some groceries? Schedule a doctor's appointment? Reply to an email? If you can't get to the big stuff on your list, focus on the small stuff, and don't forget to congratulate yourself for getting something done.

12. Hug an animal.

If you don't have a pet, can you visit a friend's? Or can you go to an animal shelter?

13. Make a "done" list instead of a "to-do" list.

Instead of overwhelming yourself right now, start feeling better about what you did get done. You can add "brushed teeth," "washed dishes," or "picked out an outfit" to your list. It doesn't matter how small the task, prove to yourself that you're effectual.

14. Watch a YouTube video that always makes you laugh

I personally recommend this one.

15. Give yourself permission to feel shitty

You're allowed to have a shitty day, and you don't have to fix it all right now. If you try to fix it and it doesn't work, that doesn't mean it's hopeless. Give yourself the time and space you need to feel what you're feeling.

16. Shut yourself off from social media or socialization for a short while

Do you get comparison syndrome, or just me? You too? Cool.
So I need to shut up social media sometimes so I'm not comparing the highlights of someone else's life, to my own life. People seem like they have it all, and they don't spend their evenings sitting in the dark, eating a whole pizza by themselves... which is not true. Other people have their own demons. You just rarely see it on social media.
I turned myself off from social media for a while, in order to help myself. I stop comparing my life to the lives of others who seem to have it all.

Chapter 22:
10 Habits of Amancio Ortega Gaona

Names like Warren Buffet and Bill Gates are household names, but do you know Amancio Ortega? Amancio is indeed one of the world's wealthiest fashion mogul. He founded Inditex, which is best known for Zara fashion and other men's and women's retail clothing, footwear, and home textiles businesses.

He is regarded as a pioneer in fast fashion thanks to his investment's eye. Zara's fashions are inspired by fashion show looks but are priced affordably to the average person. How did he get to where he is now? Here are 10 habits of Amancio Ortega.

1. **Speed Is Entirely Everything**

Ortega's "fast fashion" strategy demonstrates that speed is all you need to be ahead of your competitors and gain a market advantage. According to a business insider, a dress shown during Fashion Week can be found in Zara a few weeks later, while the same takes months to be displayed at a department store. His market aggressiveness is scheduled to design new clothes faster than anyone else in the market.

2. **Good Things Comes With Patience**

Although ten years may seem interminable when starting a business, it pays off. Being patient allows you to wait, observe, and decide when it is appropriate to act. It was after Zara went international 10 years later after trying different business approaches that Ortega broke through. Accordingly, all you need to do is take a step back, regroup, and look for better solutions.

3. **It is About What Customers Want**

Ortega's fashion sense stems from his observation of what people wear and listening to what they want. As his guiding business model, he does not base his inventory on runway shows but rather on what customers want. The customer must remain your primary focus, both in developing your new designs and the related activities.

4. **Introverts Are Also Entrepreneurs**

Many successful entrepreneurs, such as Ortega, are not extroverts, as might be expected in their line of work. Ortega once stated that even if you aren't the party's life, you can still run a successful business. He is the type of person who avoids speaking to the press at all costs, so little is known about him.

5. **Be Modest and Humble**

Ortega's journey is a classic rags-to-riches story, but he has remained true to his humble beginnings. He dropped out of school to start making money. According to The Telegraph, he has never had an office because he prefers working very close with his employees. A humble beginning does not preclude you from becoming successful, and success does not preclude you from remaining modest and humble. Those qualities can be extremely beneficial in both your personal and professional life.

6. Keep On Innovating

As Ortega puts it, "the worst thing you can do is becoming self-satisfied." Success is never guaranteed, so don't be satisfied with what you've already done. If you want to innovate, don't be concerned more with the outcome than the process.

7. Maintain Control Over Supply Chain

When you focus on a specific supply chain, you will undoubtedly respond to new trends accordingly. While many fashion companies stock clothing made in China due to low labor costs, Inditex sources most of its products from Spain, Portugal, and Morocco, according to The Economist in 2012. Ortega's stores only sell what customers want, so there are no unsold items.

8. Keep in Mind What Motivates You

Remembering what makes you wake up early in the morning to do what you do is your drive for success. Take, for instance, Ortega's childhood; he witnessed his mother being denied credit at a grocery store when he was young. At this moment, he was motivated to start working right away so that his family wouldn't have to be in such a situation again.

9. Age Is Not a Limit to Success

Sometimes you're led to believe that you must be successful at a young age, much like Steve Jobs or Mark Zuckerberg. However, Ortega founded Zara when he was nearly 40 years old. While that isn't particularly old by most people's standards, it isn't your typical twenty- or thirty-something millionaire story. It's reassuring to know that it's never too late to pursue your dreams and ambitions, as Ortega did.

10. Enjoy the Finer Things in Life

Despite his modesty and humbleness, Ortega also engages in some fun activities. He spends his free time horse riding and owns a horse riding center in Finisterre, Spain. He also owns a high-end Audi A8 sedan. It's okay to have time for yourself; spend money vacationing if you can afford it.

Conclusion

Amancio Ortega Gaona's success story is truly inspiring, as he rose from nothing to become one of Europe's richest businessmen and fashion pioneers. No matter small you start, you'll surely reach there. But only if you're motivated enough to see it.

Chapter 23:
Treat Failure Like A Scientist

Have you ever studied the life of a scientist in general? Do you know what a scientist actually does? A scientist conducts experiments to study the true nature and the working of the universe.

Scientists have a strategy to work ahead. They perform the experiments and they get results. Some are in the favor of their original theory and some are against them.

But never do these results have a personal attachment to anything. The results are data points and each data point has an importance to the study.

The scientist cannot neglect any result whether it be a success or a total failure because it will make them realize the faults they made the first time and will eventually help them and others after them to take a better start or a better theory.

The same is the case with our lives. We have to understand the working philosophy of life and failures.

People get carried away with the smallest of setbacks. We get discouraged and demotivated by the smallest of things that might not even be that big a deal. But we are so used to making such a big deal out of every little hitch.

We get stuck in the pitfall that we create ourselves and never try to realize the true mercy or lesson that little moments of pain and failure might have taught us.

Failures leave a mark, that is for sure. But those marks don't have to be bad. Whether you make those marks a war wound or a scar is up to you.

You live life as you please. Other people do the same thing. But we are not all the same, and no one can say what is right and what is wrong. But there is a simple way to judge. Let's say we get a reward for doing something good and it makes us feel good.

But when we do something from the top of our head and we are not sure what impact it will have on others, the result will make it clear and will be a lesson for the rest of our lives.

Your intentions are always in the right place, but failures still get you. So failing is not fun, but it should be held against you. You had a reason for all of this and now you have a reason to not do the same thing again.

This result made you eliminate one small thing that made you look bad the first time. So you were able to remove one more spot from your bigger picture and now you are a better individual altogether.

Failure is simply a cost you have to pay on the way to being right. Your failures don't define you, but you can define your failures. You can either let it remain a failure or you can change it into a success story by sticking to the process of turning wrongs into rights. And you will go through this learning throughout your life.

Chapter 24:
Make Your Life Better By Saying 'Thank You'

We are an ungrateful species. We are not grateful enough for what we have on our plates or for what someone else does for it. Even if we are on the receiving end of it, we don't appreciate it much.

We think that the word 'Thank you should be reserved for a very special moment. We treat it as if it is a very posh word and can't be used in many instances. But the reality is that we are not grateful enough to have the courage to thank more than we are doing right now.

You are not losing anything and it certainly doesn't affect your image in others' eyes. It surely helps to get things done more easily and quickly if you were to thank more often. It would help you get a better place in others' judgment of you and it would help you fit in with anyone.

Let's say you were to receive congrats for any of your achievements from any of your colleagues. Would it be rude if you weren't to return the compliment with a simple 'Thank You'?

Wouldn't you be called an egotistical person for not even appreciating the other with a simple compliment?

What if you were to say 'Thank You' for even the smallest of virtues happening to you? You would be praised for your gratitude towards others and you would be celebrated even more for even your smallest achievements.

You not only have to thank the people around you, but you should also thank god or your luck or your life for every moment that led you to this day.

Thank you for the hard times that made you appreciate the good times. Thank you for the lessons that you needed for you personal development. Thank you for a healthy life. Thank you for all the energies that drive me. Thank you for the drive. Thank you for the confidence. Thank you for my spirit. Thank you for the courage to keep me going through the hard times. Thank you for everything that we take for granted.

You should thank the people in your life that make your life worth living for. Thank them more than often because they have done a lot for you and also thank them for everything they will do for you in the future.

It won't hurt you to be grateful to others and it won't make anyone want you less. It will only increase your importance in others' life and them wanting to do more for you.

Take some time out of your life every day and just run your whole day like a flashback. Concentrate on the moments of respect and kindness that you received from anyone. Take some time out the next day and just go and thank them all. You would be surprised by what you receive from them, and what it makes you feel for yourself. Your trust in humanity will be immortal with this simple habit!

Chapter 25:
10 Habits Of Happy People

Happiness is a state of joy. In happiness, one is thrilled, contented, and tickled by joy. It is often expressed through bursts of laughter amidst smiles and it cannot be hidden. Happiness is a state everyone desires but few can maintain. Here are ten habits of happy people:

1. They Are Outgoing

Happy people are very social. They easily interact with strangers and make friends faster than ordinary people. They are charming to a fault and you cannot help but love their company.

Happy people are easily noticeable in a room full of different people. They are conspicuously outgoing to initiate trips, vacations, and team-building activities. Their social nature makes them thrive both in outdoor and indoor interactions.

2. They Are Self-Driven

Happy people have a strong personality that drives them in life. They are not coerced to do something and often act out of self-will. They stand out from a population that requires much convincing before they act.

They live a purposeful life that is crystal in their minds. Happy people do not need an external influence to be happy. They genuinely derive pleasure from what they do.

3. They Wake Up Early

Happy people know the secret of waking up early and do not need persuasion to wake up earlier than everybody else.
In waking up early, they keep off conflict with other people who could ruin their day. They build the foundation of the day ahead of them in the morning and they can maintain the tempo until the end. Strangers can do very little to ruin their happiness.

4. They Are Positive About Life

Happy people are very optimistic about life. Positivity is their middle name. They hardly entertain thoughts of failure. Like all of us, happiness is a choice they have to constantly make and work towards it. It distinguishes them from everyone else.
How can you be happy if you do not see the good out of the ugly? Happy people look at the brighter side of life because the grass is not greener on the other side but where you water it.

5. They Keep The Company Of Other Happy People

Happy people keep the fire of happiness burning because they associate with like-minded people. They share ideas and strategies on how to pursue their purpose. They also encourage each other when hope is bleak.
The company of sad and angry people is devastating because it gives no room for happiness to thrive. Happy people embrace each other's company because it is all they have got if they are to stay happy.

6. They Read Success Stories

Success stories are inspiring. They make us pull our socks and give us hope to succeed as others have. Happy people read and share success stories because therein lies happiness. They bask in the glory of their friends because they believe their turn too shall come.

Happy people shun bad news and stories of despair because they are discouraging and one could succumb to depression if they are not careful.

7. They Know How To Handle Bad News And Rejection

Happy people know that rejection does not spell doom for them. They have hope that they can rise above all challenges they face and still be happy. Unlike ordinary people who take rejection personally and despair, happy people consider it as another phase of life.

Handling bad news is a skill that happy people have perfected. Although some bad news could hit them hard, they know how to soak in their happiness and not live in sadness.

8. They Are Agents Of Change

Happy people are agents of change wherever they go. They make a difference with their speech and their aura changes everything. Everybody can feel the impact of happy people wherever they are.

Happy people inspire others to be like them. They recruit others in their league of happiness because they desire to see a changing world.

9. They Are Loving And Caring

Happy people can afford to be caring because they have no traces of bitterness or anger within them. They genuinely care for the welfare of other people.

Happiness makes people loving unlike those who harbor anger. You can only give what you have and it is natural for happy people to care more and sad people hurt more.

10. They Live An Authentic Lifestyle

Authenticity is a mark of happy people. They live a genuine lifestyle without seeking to impress anyone. Their joy does not lie in the approval of strangers but the satisfaction of their needs.

Happy people live within their financial means and not in the standards that other people have put for them. Their priorities are independent of external influence.

In conclusion, happy people are easy to spot. It is everybody's dream to be happy but a very elusive one. These ten habits of happy people distinguish them from others.

Chapter 26:
Happy People are Okay with Not Being Okay

All of us have a tendency where we constantly try to make people feel better about ourselves. We are fundamentally driven by empathy and compassion but what happens often is that these two are misdirected. Then we put our idea of okay onto other people and ourselves. Have you ever wondered what would it feel like when we simply whatever comes our way? When we are physically sick, of course, we take medicines to feel better, but there are also times when we are in emotional pain, and then we have no medicine to take and what happens is we seek out a solution, and that puts off the process where we can feel our feelings.

If you go through a breakup and do not allow yourself to feel the pain, what you will do is harm the next person you will date or sabotage your relationship with them. What will heal your wound is actively processing your emotions. This is not at all going to be comfortable, but it is essential for your emotional growth. What you need to do is start shedding the shame that surrounds not being okay. Just because you are in pain and not at the top of your work does not mean that you are weak. You also need to know that you are not the only one who thinks like that. We have been conditioned in this way of dysfunctional thinking and feeling. Most of us think that this is normal and normal is fine, but if you talk about health, that is a different story.

Of course, there are actions that you take that help you release the emotional pain you are in, but you have to remember that almost all of these actions will ask you to focus on yourself before you start focusing on others—for example, yoga. Yoga teaches you that your pain is not permanent, and it also tells us about how we have to be in an uncomfortable pose for a while to release that pain.

You have to remember that the only focus over here is you and you alone, but because we are all on a journey, we do get wind up in others' problems, which helps us find profound connections with them. It is okay to feel scared, or to feel pain, to feel uncertain, to feel lonely, to feel grief, it is okay to not be okay, and these are some of the things that you should never forget.

All the pain that you are feeling right now is not permanent. It will eventually pass. What you can do is honour your emotional experience by not avoiding it and being present for it; you should not try to distract yourself with every fibre of your being. This is a process that will help you heal and grow and move forward on this road. Show up for whatever you feel, even if it is just for a day.

Chapter 27:
6 Ways To Attract Anything You Want In Life

It is common human nature that one wants whatever one desires in life. People work their ways to get what they need or want. This manifestation of wanting to attract things is almost in every person around us. A human should be determined to work towards his goal or dreams through sheer hard work and will. You have to work towards it step by step because no matter what we try or do, we will always have to work for it in the end. So, it is imperative to work towards your goal and accept the fact that you can't achieve it without patience and dedication.

We have to start by improving ourselves day by day. A slight change a day can help us make a more considerable change for the future. We should feel the need to make ourselves better in every aspect. If we stay the way we are, tomorrow, we will be scared of even a minor change. We feel scared to let go of our comfort zone and laziness. That way, either we or our body can adapt to the changes that make you better, that makes you attract better.

1. **Start With Yourself First**

We all know that every person is responsible for his own life. That is why people try to make everything revolves around them. It's no secret that everyone wants to associate with successful, healthy, and charming people. But, what about ourselves? We should also work on ourselves to become the person others would admire. That is the type of person people love. He can also easily attract positive things to himself. It becomes easier to be content with your desires. We need to get ourselves together and let go of all the things we wouldn't like others doing.

2. **Have A Clear Idea of Your Wants**

Keeping in mind our goal is an easy way to attract it. Keep reminding yourself of all the pending achievements and all the dreams. It helps you work towards it, and it enables you to attract whatever you want. Make sure that you are aware of your intentions and make them count in your lives. You should always make sure to have a crystal-clear idea of your mindset, so you will automatically work towards it. It's the most basic principle to start attracting things to you.

3. **Satisfaction With Your Achievements**

It is hard to stop wanting what you once desired with your heart, but you should always be satisfied with anything you are getting. This way, when you attract more, you become happier. So, it is one of the steps to draw things, be thankful. Be thankful for what you are getting and what you haven't. Every action has a reason for itself. It doesn't mean just to let it be. Work for your goals but also acknowledge the ones already achieved by you in life. That way you will always be happy and satisfied.

4. **Remove Limitations and Obstacles**

We often limit ourselves during work. We have to know that there is no limit to working for what you want when it comes to working for what you want. You remove the obstacles that are climbing their way to your path. It doesn't mean to overdo yourselves, but only to check your capability. That is how much pressure you can handle and how far you can go in one go. If you put your boundaries overwork, you will always do the same amount, thus, never improving further. Push yourself a little more each time you work for the things you want in life.

5. **Make Your Actions Count**

We all know that visualizing whatever you want makes it easier to get. But we still cannot ignore the fact that it will not reach us unless we do some hard work and action. Our actions speak louder than words, and they speak louder than our thoughts. So, we have to make sure that our actions are built of our brain image. That is the way you could attract the things you want in life. Action is an essential rule for attracting anything you want in life.

6. Be Optimistic About Yourselves

Positivity is an essential factor when it comes to working towards your goals or dreams. When you learn to be optimistic about almost everything, you will notice that everything will make you satisfied. You will attract positive things and people. Negative vibes will leave you disappointed in yourself and everyone around you. So, you will have to practice positivity. It may not be easy at first while everyone around you is pushing you to negativity. That is where your test begins, and you have to prove yourself to them and yourself. And before you know it, you are attracting things you want.

Conclusion

Everyone around us wants to attract what they desire, but you have to start with yourself first. You only have to focus on yourself to achieve what you want. And attracting things will come naturally to you. Make sure you work for your dreams and goals with all your dedication and determination. With these few elements, you will be attracting anything you want.

Chapter 28:
Saying Yes To Things

Today we're going to talk about why saying yes can be a great thing for you and why you should do so especially in social invites.

Life you see is a funny thing. As humans, we tend to see things one dimensionally. And we tend to think that we have a long life ahead of us. We tend to take things for granted. We think we will have time to really have fun and relax after we have retired and so we should spend all our efforts and energy into building a career right now, prioritising it above all else. When faced with a choice between work and play, sometimes many of us, including myself choose work over social invites.

There were periods in my life that i routinely chose work over events that it became such a habit to say no. Especially as an entrepreneur, the interaction between colleagues or being in social events is almost reduced to zero. It became very easy and comfortable to live in this bubble where my one and only priority in life is to work work work. 24 hours, 7 days a week. Of course, in reality a lot of time was wasted on social media and Netflix, but u know, at least i could sort of pretend that i was kind of working all day. And I was sort of being productive and sort of working towards my goals rather than "wasting time on social events". That was what I told myself anyway.

But life does not work that way. As I prioritised work over all else, soon all the social invite offers started drying up. My constant "nos" were becoming evident to my social circle and I was being listed as perpetually unavailable or uninterested in vesting time or energy into any friendships or relationships. And as i retreated deeper and deeper into this black hole of "working remotely" i found myself completely isolated from new experiences and meeting new people, or even completely stopped being involved in any of my friend's lives.

I've successfully written myself out of life and I found myself all alone in it.

Instead of investing time into any meaningful relationships, I found that my closest friends were my laptop, tablet, phone, and television. Technology became my primary way of interacting with the world. And I felt connected, yet empty. I was always plugged in to wifi, but i lived my life through a screen instead of my own two eyes. My work and bedroom became a shell of a home that I spent almost all my time, and life just became sort of pointless. And I just felt very alone.

As I started to feel more and more like something was missing, I couldn't quite make out what it was that led me to this feeling. I simply though to myself, hey I'm prioritising work and my career, making money is what the internet tells me I should do, and not having a life is simply part of the price you have to pay... so why am I so incredibly unhappy?

As it turns out, as I hope many of you have already figured out at this point, that life isn't really just about becoming successful financially. While buying a house, getting a car, and all that good stuff is definitely something that we should strive towards, we should not do so at the expense of our friends. That instead of saying no to them, we should start saying yes, at least once in a while. We need to signal to our friends that hey, yes even though I'm very busy, but I will make an effort to carve out time for you, so that you know I still value you in my life and that you are still a priority.

We need to show our friends that while Monday may not work for us, that I have an opening maybe 2 weeks later if you're still down. That we are still available to grow this friendship.

I came to a point in my life where I knew something had to change. As I started examining my life and the decisions I had made along the way with regards to my career, I knew that what I did wrong was saying no WAAAAAY too often. As I tried to recall when was the last time I actually when I went out with someone other than my one and only BFF, I simply could not. Of the years that went by, I had either said that I was too busy, or even on the off chances that I actually agreed to some sort of meetup, I had the habit of bailing last minute on lunch and dinner appointments with friends. And I never realized that i had such a terrible reputation of being a flaker until I started doing some serious accounting of my life. I had become someone that I absolutely detested without even realising it. I have had people bail on me at the very last minute before, and I hated that feeling. And whenever someone did that to me, I generally found it difficult to ask them out again because I felt that they weren't really that interested in meeting me anyway. That they didn't even bother to reschedule the appointment. And little did I know, I was becoming that very same person and doing the very thing that I hate to my friends. It is no wonder that I started dropping friends like flies with my terrible actions.

As I came to this revelation, I started panicking. It was as if a truck had hit me so hard that I felt that I was in a terrible accident. That how did I let myself get banged up to that extent?

I started scrolling through my contact lists, trying to find friends that might still want to hang out with me. I realized that my WhatsApp was basically dry as a desert, and my calendar was just work for the last 3 years straight with no meaningful highlights, no social events worth noting.

It was at this point that I knew I had made a huge mistake and I needed to change course immediately. Salvaging friendships and prioritising social activities went to the top of my list.

I started creating a list of friends that I had remotely any connection to in the last 5 years and I started asking them out one by one. Some of my friends who i had asked out may not know this, but at that point in my life, i felt pretty desperate and alone and I hung on to every meeting as if my life depended on it. Whilst I did manage to make some appointments and met up with some of them. I soon realized that the damage had been done. That my friends had clearly moved on without me... they had formed their own friends at work and elsewhere, and I was not at all that important to have anymore. It was too little too late at that point and there was not much I could do about it. While I made multiple attempts to ask people out, I did not receive the same offers from people. It felt clearly like a one-way street and I felt that those people that I used to call friends, didn't really see me as one. You see growing a friendship takes time, sometimes years of consistent meetups before this person becomes indispensable in your life. Sharing unique experiences that allow your friends to see that you are truly vested in them and that you care about them and want to spend time with them. I simply did not give myself that chance to be integrated into someone's life in that same way, I did not invest that time to growing those friendships and I paid the price for it.

But I had to learn all these the hard way first before I can receive all the good that was about to come in the future.

Chapter 29:
How To Stop Being A Narcissist

Narcissists often get flak for being incapable of change.

The reason, according to psychologists, is that most narcissists aren't really aware of their narcissistic tendencies. These issues are often deep-seated, and self-preservation stops them from even recognizing their problems.

But chances are, if you're reading this, you're one of those who want to change. Admitting you might have Narcissistic Personality Disorder is already a step forward.

Self-aware narcissists can change. In this article, we've curated seven key steps on how to stop being a narcissist, according to some of the world's top psychology experts. We then go through the negative impacts of narcissism, followed by a discussion on whether narcissists can really change.

You have Narcissistic Personality Disorder if you:

- Think quite highly of yourself, like you're the only important person in the world.
- Are self-entitled and feel that you deserve nothing but the best.
- Demand recognition even if you didn't do anything to deserve it.
- Exaggerate your skills and achievements and brag about them excessively.
- Make everything about you.
- Use and manipulate people to get what you want.

- Unwilling to recognize and value the needs of others.

Overcoming narcissism is no simple process. Absolute change may be near impossible. However, you can make changes that will create a positive impact on your life.

Know what your "triggers" are: Narcissistic behaviour often emerges when a person suffering from Narcissistic Personality Disorder gets "triggered."

According to Greenberg, "triggers" are: "…situations, words, or behaviours that arouse strong negative feelings in you. People with narcissistic issues tend to overreact when they are "triggered" and do things that they later regret."

As a first step, it's important to know in which situations your narcissism comes out. Learning what they are can help you identify the reasons behind your narcissism, so you may be able to handle them accordingly.

For example, if you experience narcissistic tendencies and want to become aware of your triggers, you may notice that you often feel a surge of anger when someone you perceive being of a "lower status" challenges your authority in the workplace

Or you may notice that you are often dismissive of other people when they suggest ideas.

Whatever your particular triggers are, start to take note of them. It may be useful to carry a notebook with you or jot them down in a note-taking app on your phone.

Over time, you'll start to notice patterns on when you feel triggered by others and react with narcissistic tendencies.

Manage your impulses: Narcissist people are often impulsive and make decisions without thinking of the consequences. If you display narcissist tendencies, it's important to emphasize thinking first and reacting later.

According to Greenberg: "Practice inhibiting or delaying your normal response when triggered. Your 'normal' response is the now unwanted one that you do automatically. It has become wired as a habit into the neurons of your brain."

The key step to changing your behaviours is to become aware of your impulses. This gives you the opportunity to create behavioural change in your life.

Taking note of your triggers as recommended in step one will teach you to create some space between the stimulus of the trigger and your response. Pausing when triggered opens up the opportunity to create a new set of behaviours

Chapter 30:
10 Habits of Mukesh Ambani

From managing his father-founded company to becoming India's most affluent and business tycoon, Mukesh Ambani knows, thinks, and does certain things which you don't. Mukesh chairs and runs multi-billion Reliance Industries, which accounts for a hefty 5percent of India's GDP. Without a doubt, he's indeed leading a very successful and wealthy life.

If you were to ask Mukesh Ambani about his rise to success, he would have to speak from years of experience. But, because he's a guru, not just a "talker," he believes that whatever comes of you is a direct result of your understanding of the nature of your business. So, what is his path to success?

Here are 10 habits of Mukesh Ambani.

1. Speak Less, Do More

Israel More's quote "talk less, do more" perfectly describes Mukesh's approach to progress. He not only keeps small social circles, but he also avoids scandals as much as possible. He's the type of person who will advise you to stand your ground by focusing on your business and possibly avoid politicking. Despite being India's most talked-about business personality, he does not promote or stimulate the attention he receives.

2. Treat the Investor's Money With Caution

Ambani believes that you should treat your investors' money with more care than your own. It's a chicken and egg situation, but it appears to go hand in hand with high investor confidence. It is unknown whether his success came before his special handling of investors' money. Still, he is the polar opposite of how many businesses treat the investment as if they have hit the lottery.

3. Money Is the By-Product of Success

Most successful people, including Musk and Jack Ma, have talked against holding money-driven motivation when carrying on your business. Accordingly, Mukesh's father also believed that chasing money won't guarantee success. He founded Reliance with the same thought, which Mukesh carried on after taking over, and he's now reaping the benefits.

4. Dream Big

Dreaming big goes hand in hand with working hard to make it a reality. Words may ring dull, but how can a business materialize without a vision and a plan to guide it? As Mukesh stated during his "Global Living Legends" acceptance speech, "align your passion with your life goal and pursue the goal with excellence, and success will chase you."

5. Nurture Your Staff, Not the Profits

Ambani has primarily built his company by taking the bold step of assembling the right team. He believes in an organizational culture that demonstrates empathy, fosters trust and relationships, and views mistakes as learning opportunities. To bring out the best in your employees, create a work environment that nurtures their skills and talents. And you can only do this if you prioritize employees over profits.

6. Credibility Conveys a High Premium

Ambani advises on being there whenever it is your team that needs you or the competition. Recognize, innovate, and plan for the future. He believes that, in addition to cash inflow and outflow, credibility must be protected.

7. Risks Give the Most Vital Insights

Sometime back in 2015, Ambani made a risky decision, which many thought was too risky. That is, his decision to roll out 4G; yes, you read that correctly! 4G is a mobile phone network. He once said that if you do not take risks, you will not experience significant growth in your life. And, yes, he proved this throughout his career.

8. See Everyone as a Potential Customer

According to Ambani's target market strategy, a billion people means a billion potential customers. There is no way he will let customers slip through his reach, thus taking the chance to generate value for them and, in return, making something for himself. When you consider how populated India is, you can see the volumes business people in this part of the world have to sell.

9. Trust All, but Rely on No One

Ambani believes in being your drive to succeed. Yes, you will need to be around people, but you need not rely on anyone but yourself for business success. While he has a trusted team of a few people who have played critical roles in expanding his empire, Ambani understands that nothing beats perseverance and self-learning. Trust is important, but you must keep abreast of all types of emergencies that keep the company running.

10. Trust Your Gut Instincts

There have been several controversies concerning Mukesh, 'a rich man without a heart' owing to his splurging money on building his house and investing in the IPL cricket team. However, Mukesh does what he deems suitable, and most of it turns out to be "right thing to do" for him. Follow your instincts and disregard anyone's opinion especially when it doesn't add value to you, and because haters are always a mile away.

Conclusion

What more! He is the perfect example of a businessman who has his way with business. Undoubtedly, Mukesh has achieved a lot in his field because of his determination, hard work, and willpower.

Chapter 31:
When It Is Time To Let Go and Move On (Career)

Today we're going to talk about a topic that I hope will motivate you to quit that job that you hate or one that you feel that you have nothing more to give anymore.

For the purpose of this video, we will focus mainly on career as I believe many of you may feel as though you are stuck in your job but fear quitting because you are afraid you might not find a better one.

For today's topic, I want to draw attention to a close friend of mine who have had this dilemma for years and still hasn't decided to quit because he is afraid that he might not get hired by someone else.

In the beginning of my friend's career, he was full of excitement in his new job and wanted to do things perfectly. Things went pretty smoothly over the course of the first 2 years, learning new things, meeting new friends, and getting settled into his job that he thought he might stay on for a long time to come seeing that it was the degree that he had pursued in university. However when the 3rd year came along, he started to feel jaded with his job. Everyday he would meet ungrateful and sometimes mean customers who were incredibly self-entitled. They would be rude and he started dreading going to work more and more each day. This aspect of the job wore him down and he started to realise that he wasn't happy at all with his work.

Having had a passion for fitness for a while now, he realized that he felt very alive when he attended fitness classes and enjoyed working out and teaching others how to work out. He would fiddle with the idea of attending a teacher training course that would allow him to be a professional and certified fitness coach.

As his full time job started to become more of a burden, he became more serious about the prospect of switching careers and pursuing a new one entirely. At his job, realized that the company wasn't generous at all with the incentives and gruelling work hours, but he stayed on as he was afraid he wouldn't find another job in this bad economy. The fear was indeed real so he kept delaying trying to quit his job. Before he knew it 3 years more had passed and by this time he full on dreaded every single minute at his job.

It was not until he made that faithful decision one day to send in his resignation letter and to simultaneously pay for the teacher training course to become a fitness instructor did his fortunes start to change for him. The fortunes in this wasn't about money. It was about freedom. It was about growth. And it was about living.

We all know deep in our hearts when it is time to call it quits to something. When we know that there is nothing more that we can possibly give to our job. That no amount of time more could ever fulfill that void in us. That we just simply need to get out and do something different.

You see, life is about change. As we grow, our priorities change, our personalities change, our expectations change, and our passions and our interests change as well. If we stay in one place too long, especially in a field or in something that we have hit a wall at, we will feel stuck, and we will feel dread. We will feel that our time spent is not productive and we end up feeling hopeless and sorry for ourselves.

Instead when we choose to let go, when we choose to call time on something, we open up the doors for time on other ventures, and other adventures. And our world becomes brighter again.

I challenge each and everyone of you to take a leap of faith. You know deep in your hearts when it is time to move on from your current job and find the next thing. If you dont feel like you are growing, or if you feel that you absolutely hate your job because there is no ounce of joy that you can derive from it, move on immediately. Life is too short to be spending 10 hours of your life a day on something that you hate, that sucks the living soul out of you. Give yourself the time and space to explore, to find some other path for you to take. You will be surprised what might happen when you follow your heart.

Chapter 32:
How To Improve Your Communication Skills

Today we're going to talk about a topic that could help you be a better communicator with your spouse, your friends, and even your colleagues and bosses. Being able to express yourself fluently and eloquently is a skill that is incredibly important as it allows us to express our thoughts and ideas freely and fluently in ways that others might understand.

When we are able to communicate easily with others, we are able to build instant rapport with them and this allows us to appear better than we actually are. We may be able to cover some of our flaws if we are able to communicate our strengths better.

So how do we actually become better communicators? I believe that the easiest way to begin is to basically start talking with more people. It is my experience that after spending much time on my own without much social interaction, that i saw my standard of communication dropped quite drastically. You see, being able to talk well is essentially a social skill, and without regular practice and use, you just simply can't improve it. I saw that with irregular use of social interaction, the only skill that actually improved for me was texting. And we all know that texting is a very impersonal way to communicate and does not actually translate to real world fluency in person to person conversations.

Similarly, watching videos on communication and reading tips and tricks really does not help at all unless you apply it in the real world. And to have regular practice, you need to start by either inviting all your friends out to a meal so that you can strike up conversations and improve from there, or by maybe joining a social interaction group class of sorts that would allow you to practice verbal communication skills. If u were to ask me, I believe that making the effort to speak to your friends and colleagues is the best way to begin. And you can even ask them for feedback if there are any areas that they find you could improve on. Expect genuine feedback and criticisms as they go if you hope to improve, and do not take them personally.

It is with my personal experience that i became extremely rusty when it came to talking to friends at one point in my life, when i was sort of living in isolation. I find it hard to connect even with my best friend, and i found it hard to find topics to discuss about, mainly because i wasn't really living much to begin with, and there was nothing i was experiencing in life that was really worth sharing. If you stop living life, you stop having significant moments, you stop having problems that need solving, and you stop having friends that needs supporting. I believe the best way is to really try to engage the person you are talking to by asking them very thoughtful questions and by being genuinely interested in what they have to say. Which also coincidentally ties into my previous video about being a good listener. which you should definitely check out if you haven't done so already.

Being a good listener is also a big part of being a good communicator. The other part being able to respond in a very insightful way that isn't patronising. We can only truly connect with the person we are talking to if we are able to first understand on an empathetic level, what they are going through, and then to reply with the same level of compassion and empathy that they require of us.

With colleagues and bosses, we should be able to strike up conversations that are professional yet natural. And being natural in the way we communicate takes practice from all the other social interactions that precede us.

I believe that being a good communicator really takes time and regular practice in order for it to come one day and just click for us. For a start, just simply try to be friendly and place yourself out of your comfort zone, only then can you start to see improvements.

I challenge each and everyone of you today who are striving to be better communicators to start asking out your friends and colleagues for coffees and dinners. Get the ball rolling and just simply start talking. Over time, it will just come naturally to you. Trust me.

Chapter 33:
9 Signs You're Feeling Insecure About a Relationship

Being in a new relationship is often the most exciting part. You go back and forth with your date, wondering if he or she likes you, and you play the dating game as all new romance starts out. But what happens when you start to fall for someone more than you thought you would have liked to at this stage.

It is never a pleasant feeling for us to feel that we are not in control, but that is the process of being vulnerable and admitting to yourself that you do have a personal investment in this relationship. If you are unsure about what you are going through,

Here are 7 Signs That Show You Are Feeling Insecure About A Relationship:

1. You Start Checking Their "Last Seen"

We have all done this before - We wonder why it takes so long for the person to reply our texts so we check our messaging apps constantly to check when they were last online. We then draw deductions that they may have deliberately chosen not to reply to our messages despite being online. However unhealthy habit of checking their "last seen" only takes power away from our self-worth. We need to stop obsessing over such small little details and just focus on the things we are supposed to do for the day. If the person genuinely likes you, he or she will find the time to reply in a thoughtful and appropriate manner.

2. You Anxiously Hope That They Ask You Out

Waiting for the next date to happen is normal. We all expect to have some back and forth to ensure that it is not a one-sided effort in dating and relationships. However, if this becomes an anxious wait, then you might be falling into the realm of insecurity. Ideally things should happen naturally if all is going well. If you catch yourself losing sleep because he or she hasn't asked you out, take some of that power back and consider taking the initiative instead to either ask if there is going to be a next date, or even asking them out if you want to see this through. Don't let anxiety rule your dating life.

3. You Wait For Them To Say Something Sweet To Affirm Their Like of you

We all want to be woo-ed. It is a nice feeling when someone says something sweet to you just because. But if you find yourself eagerly anticipating every sentence to be something affectionate, be careful not to be disappointed if it doesn't happen ever-so-often. Dating and relationships can be a tricky business; we don't want to seem too needy or too forward at the same time. Sometimes we just have to find a balance between being overly sweet and also reserving some of it when so as not to come across too strong.

4. You Start Thinking Of The Worst-Case Scenarios

Being in the early phases of a relationship is always fun, but as the dust settles and you start thinking of the worst-case scenarios, you may be feeling insecure. We all want to go back to the part of dating where we expect nothing from the other party - we are dating a few different people at once and we have no desires to commit. But when you start catching yourself thinking of what could go wrong with someone you've decided you like more than others, it may be time to take a step back and reassess the situation. Don't jump too far ahead of the curve.

5. You Can't Focus On Your Work

Being in love and thinking about the wonderful things about the other person is a normal way to lose focus on your work. However if this lack of concentration starts revolving around worry that things could go wrong, or that the person may not like you, then you've got to snap out of it. It is never healthy to let these negative thoughts affect your daily productivity. Remember that your life always comes first - Focus on the important things and then worry about dating and relationships later.

6. You're Distraught From The Lack of Clear Signals

You find yourself second guessing everything. One minute you think your date is interested, the next you're worried he or she is not. This back and forth can take a toll on your mental capacity to handle things and you may find yourself feeling out of sorts. You wonder if your date went well or did it go disastrously. The fact that your date isn't giving you any clear signs adds to your insecurity about the whole thing.

7. You're Unsure About Where This Is Going

Similar to the previous point, this time you are unsure where this relationship is headed. Is there something there or should you cut your losses and move on. It will be hard to assess the situation and the only way to be sure is to ask him or her directly what their thoughts are about the whole matter. If they are unable to give you a clear answer, you can at least be assured that it is not all in your head. Do what is best for yourself and never be too hung up over just one person.

8. You Wonder If They Are Seeing Someone Else

This is insecurity at one of the highest levels. Trust is something that must be built over time. If you find yourself questioning whether your date or partner is seeing someone else, maybe you never really felt secure in this relationship in the first place. This could be a tricky matter to handle so once again if you find yourself doubting every aspect of this bond, maybe it's time to be dial it back until you can trust your whole heart with that person.

9. You Question Every Single Decision You Make

Second guessing ourselves and everything that we do has got to be one of the worst ways to operate in life. You question whether you said the right thing on the date, whether you made the right moves, whether you came off as confident rather weak. These are questions that we need to not bother ourselves with because it will not bring any goodness to us. Make decisions that you will stick with no matter what and stop ruminating on the past. Just do what you can now and move forward with pride.

Conclusion

Dating and relationships are not easy. It comes with its own set of rules and emotions are bound to run rampant at some point if we don't reign them in. Instead of making it harder than it already is for ourselves, simply trust that things will work out if it's meant to be. Overthinking and feeling insecure will not bring us any good. The fact is that sometimes we will get our hearts broken, but we will stand tall and learn from our past. The quest for love is not going to be a piece of cake, but if the right person comes along, things will work out.

Chapter 34:
6 Ways To Master Your Emotions

As reported by Psychology Today, psychology's answer to the question of "What is emotional mastery?" Has evolved over the last century. Early American psychology embraced the "James-Lange Theory," which held that emotions are strictly the product of physiology (a neurological response to some external stimuli). This view evolved when the "Cannon-Bard Theory" asserted that the brain's thalamus mediates between external stimuli and subjective emotional experience.

The concept of emotional mastery wasn't introduced until the 1960s with the Schachter-Singer experiment, where researchers gave participants a dose of a placebo "vitamin." Participants then watched colleagues complete a set of questionnaires. When the colleagues responded angrily to the questionnaires, the participants felt angry in turn. But when the colleagues responded happily, the participants also felt happy. The study's results implied a connection between peer influence and the felt experience of emotion.

The idea that emotions are influenced by outer as well as inner stimuli was furthered by psychiatrist Allen Beck, who demonstrated that thoughts, peer influence and circumstance shape emotions. Beck's research formed the foundation of modern-day cognitive-behavioral therapy, the gold standard of emotional mastery as it's understood today.

The Role Of Emotional Mastery In Life And Society

Feelings and emotional mastery play a role in our subjective experience and <u>interpersonal relationships</u>.

- **Emotions unify us across cultural lines**. There are six basic emotions that are universal in all cultures: happiness, sadness, fear, anger, surprise and disgust. We all experience these feelings, although there are cultural differences regarding what's an appropriate display of emotion.

- **Emotions govern our sense of well-being**. Since emotions are a product of our experiences and how we perceive those experiences, we can <u>cultivate positive emotions</u> by focusing on them. There are 10 "power emotions" that cultivate emotional mastery by creating a base of positive affect. When we incorporate even small doses of gratitude, passion, love, hunger, curiosity, <u>confidence</u>, flexibility, cheerfulness, vitality and a sense of contribution, we set the stage for feeling good about ourselves.

- **Emotional mastery supports healthy relationships**. When you're able to demonstrate emotions that are appropriate to the situation, you're able to nurture your relationships. When you don't know how to master your emotions, the opposite occurs: You might fly off the handle at minor annoyances or react with anger when sadness is a more appropriate response. Your emotional response affects those around you, which shapes your relationships for better or worse.

Learning how to master your emotions is a skill anyone can build in six straightforward steps.

1. Identify what you're really feeling

The first step in learning how to master your emotions is identifying what your feelings are. To take that step toward emotional mastery, ask yourself:

- What am i really feeling right now?
- Am i really feeling…?
- Is it something else?
-

2. Acknowledge and appreciate your emotions, knowing they support you

Emotional mastery does not mean shutting down or denying your feelings. Instead, learning how to master your emotions means appreciating them as part of yourself.

- You never want to make your emotions wrong.
- The idea that anything you feel is "wrong" is a great way to destroy honest communication with yourself as well as with others.

3. Get curious about the message this emotion is offering you

Emotional mastery means approaching your feelings with a sense of curiosity. Your feelings will teach you a lot about yourself if you let them. Getting curious helps you:

- Interrupt your current emotional pattern.
- Solve the challenge.
- Prevent the same problem from occurring in the future.

4. Get confident

The quickest and most powerful route to emotional mastery over any feeling is to remember a time when you felt a similar emotion and handled it successfully. Since you managed the emotion in the past, surely you can handle it today.

5. Get certain you can handle this not only today, but in the future as well

To master your emotions, build confidence by rehearsing handling situations where this emotion might come up in the future. See, hear and feel yourself handling the situation. This is the equivalent of lifting emotional weights, so you'll build the "muscle" you need to handle your feelings successfully.

5. Get excited and take action

Now that you've learned how to master your emotions, it's time to get excited about the fact that you can:

- Easily handle this emotion.
- Take some action right away.
- Prove that you've handled it.

Learning emotional mastery is one of the most powerful steps you can take to create a life that's authentic and fulfilling.

CPSIA information can be obtained
at www.ICGtesting.com
Printed in the USA
LVHW052228280122
709482LV00013B/390